Sex

The Complete and Effective Guide to Turning On the Passion in Couple's Sex Life.

Discover & Enjoy the Best Sex Positions

By Katy Lian

Legal Disclaimer

The information contained in this book and its contents is not designed to replace any form of medical or professional advice; and is not meant to replace the need for independent medical, financial, legal, or other professional advice or services that may be required. The content and information in this book have been provided for educational and entertainment purposes only.

The content and information contained in this book have been compiled from sources deemed reliable, and they are accurate to the best of the Author's knowledge, information, and belief.

However, the Author cannot guarantee its accuracy and validity and therefore cannot be held liable for any errors and/or omissions. Further, changes are periodically made to this book as needed. Where appropriate and/or necessary, you must consult a professional (including but not limited to your doctor, attorney, financial advisor, or other such professional) before using any of the suggested remedies, techniques, and/or information in this book.

Upon using this book's contents and information, you agree to hold harmless the Author from any damages, costs, and expenses, including any legal fees, potentially resulting from the application of any of the information in this book. This disclaimer applies to any loss, damages, or injury caused by the use and application of this book's contents, whether directly or indirectly, whether for breach of contract, tort, negligence, personal injury,

Table of Contents

Introduction

Sexual passion between a man and a woman is like fire – if you do not support it and do not refresh it with something new, it will be fading down together along with the relationship. Sex plays a deeply important role in a relationship which is more than only sexual satisfaction.

As we engage in sexual pleasure, repeating the same positions, the joy of the act fades slightly as we have nothing to look forward to except what we've already done together. To keep sex alive, partners need to mix it up a little, at the start. As couples try new and different sex positions, they will find new ways to feel erotic stimulation, and along with it, more productive ejaculations for him, and deeper and more satisfying orgasms.

There is a feeling of rapture in great sex. Exploring, and experimenting while keeping an open mind will turn up new discoveries. Trying new sexual positions has no negative effect on a partnership. On the other hand, trying and feeling wonderful in a new position is a memorable positive experience, and that will be repeated over and over.

Partners can couple in literally hundreds of positions because of our physical shape. Some positions provide for deeper penetration, while others change the angle of penetration, coming into contact with a female's G-spot.

Erogenous zones on the body are constantly being discovered through research. But the best study and most conclusive occurs in the laboratory fo the bedroom, with partners as the test subjects. Men can be stimulated in more areas than just his penis, and women can have clitoral, vaginal G-spot orgasms. Men and women often don't realize, for example, that they can achieve a vaginal orgasm, because they have never tried a sexual position that can stimulate them in a way that would help release it.

Trying new things together means couples are learning what positions can do for them at the same time. Some of the positions listed here are intensely intimate, allowing for caressing and kissing while having sexual intercourse. Others stimulate zones of erotic stimulation on the body and bring about intense sexual release, even though they are less intimate.

But couples do these together, and it only leads to a closer relationship. Great sex improves the mindset, and problems like allocating money to pay bills become less important. Day to day problems are figured out easier when partners feel close to each other and are sexually satisfied. There is both a mental and physical benefit to sex. Heart rate is regulated, and even mental health issues are mediated by intimacy and sexual release.

Chapter 1: The Positive and Negative Impact of Pornography

It's a fact that porn watching is intensely arousing. Watching attractive people copulate, perform oral sex on each other, so carefree and natural, fulfills deep desires. Fantasizing and imagining having intensely pleasurable sex with a beautiful woman or a sexy, well-endowed man, one can view, for free, any and all sex positions and wild encounters involving a couple, a threesome, and orgiastic parties that seem to be happening all around. It's inviting, encouraging the viewer to come and feel the same pleasures, live a life of daily erotic stimulation with one partner in the morning and a different partner coming over with a friend that same night.

Porn is like gambling, once started, it's very difficult to stop, even though it harms lovers and spouses, because it's so easy to be in that fantasy world. Just click a button and for hours, life is fulfilling.

Porn viewing, like actual sex, releases pleasure chemicals in the brain, and include opiate receptors. There is a real and genuine high that one feels while watching porn. The problem is that it impacts the viewer's ability to have sex. Watching too much porn makes a man unable to have sex with his girlified or his wife when he indulges too much.

The positive impact of porn as a sort of college course, is that it gives viewers inspiration to experiment, try new ways to have sex, new positions. Porn communicates the idea that it's okay to have an open mind about sex. The actors are he instructors and they demonstrate what they know before our eyes.

We get inspired (arouses) by the teacher. But then the bell rings and class are over. Walk out of the classroom (shut it off), and later on, apply what's been learned with a partner, a girlfriend, boyfriend, spouse and partner. Who knows if the porn industry encourages fidelity to a loved one? It doesn't matter because the choice to remain with some is an individual choice in the end. Realize that 99.99% of porn videos are staged. Pornographic sex is unsimulated sex, it's staged. But everything after that, the screams of ecstasy, the intense enjoyment the actors display, is, in the end, acting. After all, they call themselves "actors."

The Benefits of Sexual Exploration and Discovery

There are forces in the world who proclaim that sex is something that should be behind closed doors and should be performed only between married partners. Some even claim that sex is not to be enjoyed. People have different upbringings, and if they come from religious families, they are taught to accept that lustful thoughts are sinful thoughts. This is not a put down of religion. For many, it serves a useful function I their life. It can be positive and help the initiated have a productive life in faith.

But for someone whose success and productiveness comes from other sources, that should be accepted as well. "To each his own" and "live and let live" are good maxims to live by. If an adult wishes to try something different, he or she has that right.

Variety in sexual life is positive and healthy. Humans are creatures who have instinctual attractions and are curious about ways to enhance their sexual experience.

Chapter 2: Oral Sex Positions

Reverse Approach Cunnilingus

If your partner has been on the fence about oral sex, or she seems not to derive much pleasure from it, try this easy and comfortable position. Your mouth, lips and tongue make contact her clitoris, labia and vagina from the opposite angle.

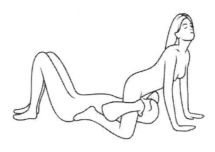

When performing this position, the man lies down on his back, and the woman straddles him from above on all fours. He takes hold of her legs by the thighs which gives him control underneath as he licks her clitoris. Lick with gentle, soft strokes to make the blood rush to her labia, making it swell.

Feeling the softness of her skin, he moves his hands and gently caress her hips while his mouth and lips move from her clitoris down to her labia. He can playfully dart his tongue in and out of her vagina, moving it back up from time to time to her clitoris. Bite her clit as well while running caressing her thighs and hips.

Next, the man moves his hands around the back of her thighs to her buttocks. He caresses and gently strokes the entrance of her ass between her butt cheeks. This area is particularly sensitive when handled gently and will increase the sensations she receives from his licking in her genital area.

When he performs the position well, she will begin to gyrate her hips, and her downward movement will allow him to stroke her belly and move up to her breasts. As his technique and he spends an adequate period of time licking her clit, moistening her vagina with his mouth and lips she'll feel an intense pleasure felt deep inside her body.

She should make sure her head is tilted back so that her hips can fall close to her partner's mouth. Her arms are straight, her palms supporting her, and her legs slightly apart, on either side of the man's head and neck. Her genitals should end up positioned about an inch (3 cm) away from her partner's mouth,

It should be noted here the importance of oral sex before coitus. When performing oral sex, the genitals are moistened on a woman, and blood flow increases to the man's penis. In addition, sexual arousal builds and builds. When partners turn to intercourse, their arousal is much more intense than it would be without oral sex. Intercourse is more intense, and couples enjoy much more powerful orgasms thanks to positions like Reverse Cowgirl.

Over time, and by doing this position more often, he will improve his technique. More satisfied, she will suggest the couple engage in this position more often before intercourse.

Fellatio - Man on Top

This male-dominant position is another "prelude to penetration" sex position. The opposite of the typical oral sex position, in this scenario the man is on top and the woman at bottom.

When she is on top, she has complete control as the man lies supine on his back. She is able to stroke his penis, put it in her mouth and take it out when she wishes, as he enjoys her attentiveness to his genitals.

The Man on Top position turns control completely over to him. Now he is on top and she is underneath, lying down below him. However, she is not completely supine. Her head is raised, and he straddles his legs on either side of her thighs.

To perform this unique and satisfying position (especially for him), the woman raises her head and takes hold of him and grasps the sides of his back. As soon as the couple is ready, he inserts his erect penis down into her mouth.

The Man on Top position is most satisfying when a rhythm is established between the partners. He starts slowly, thrusting into her mouth and establishing the same slow rhythm that occurs during intercourse. Her head moves forward when he thrusts into her mouth, and back out when he moves away. When the couple moves closer and away simultaneously, a perfect rhythm is established.

Throughout this position, he rests his weight on the palms of his hands. He can, if able, place one of his hands on the back of her head and push her head towards his penis. However, this will not be necessary if she has a firm enough hold of his back.

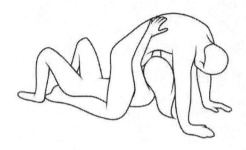

Unlike the girl on top oral sex position, she is unable to use her hands because she is grasping him to maintain support. Only her mouth is involved.

His penis goes deeper into her mouth because of the angle of his penetration. The feeling for him is highly satisfying because the feeling for him is like vaginal penetration. It is a "same but different' kind of feeling. Fr him, being on top and possessing control of her and his movement, arousal is highly likely for him.

Women can feel gratified that their role is pleasing him. If rhythm is well-established and she can take his penis deeper into her mouth, then she has been successful.

This level of difficulty in performing this position is "Medium" because the man needs to have more strength in his shoulders and arms. For the woman, unless her partner supports her head by gripping the back, she has to possess more strength in her back and shoulders to withstand a lengthy scene.

Couples can discuss before engaging in Man on Top what to do if the man becomes so aroused that he can ejaculate. They should agree on what will happen next. Will he pull out? Will he pull out and spray on her breasts and body? Or ejaculate on her face? Will she allow him to come in her mouth?

Standing Oral Sex

The Standing Oral Sex is an exhilaratingly different way to perform oral sex. This approach should be performed when couples are feeling energetic due to the physical requirements the position calls for.

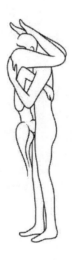

He stands and picks up the female and turns her upside down to where her mouth is near his penis and his mouth is in contact with her labia, vagina and clitoris. He wraps his arms around her just above the buttocks and she grips him on his back above his buttocks. His head is between her legs.

This position is stimulating because of the direct angles of each partner's mouths on their partner's genitals. The woman can take more of the man's penis into her mouth. He can reach with his tongue the female's clitoris, labia and vagina. Also, the thrill of being lifted and working against gravity makes this position memorable.

69 Sex Position

This non-coitus position is referred to as "69" due to the carnal configuration that allows males and females to give each other simultaneous oral sex. When partners match their mouths to each other's genitals, it appears visually like the number 69.

This position has become popular to the satisfaction it gives both partners, and it is a wonderful position to do before penetrative sex. Both partners lie down without any discomfort, allowing them to focus on pleasuring the other while they themselves are feeling pleasurable sensations.

69 makes a man harder prior to intercourse and makes a woman's vagina wet in preparation for sex. It also allows for each partner to wrap their arms around each other and hold each other close as they lick and suck each other. Because 69 moistens the vagina, it is not necessary to use lube if the man has a large penis or if intercourse is painful.

There are several positions in which you can perform the 69-sex position. If she is on top of him, she can control how much pressure she receives. She straddles his chest, facing his toes, leans forward and straightens out her legs. This gives her easy access to his genitals, also giving him easy access to hers.

Another variation is to have him place his head slightly over the edge of the bed, widthwise, while the woman stands above him with her legs spread enough for his head to fit between. The woman leans forward and sucks on his penis. The man at this angle can lick further down between the woman's legs, giving her a unique and stimulating feeling.

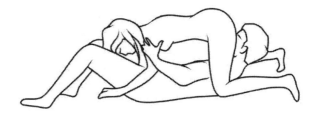

Another way to start is for the woman to lean over and kiss the man's mouth, then crawl over him onto the bed, licking him on the way down from his chest all the way to his groin until both partners have mouth to genitals contact.

If being on top is tiring for her, she can lie back and let him straddle her. An advantage to this approach is it allows the woman to titillate the man by fondling his shaft, testicles and his perineum (between his butt and testicles which is full of nerve endings to stimulate with the tongue). IN this position she gives heightened pleasure to her partner.

The couple can lie sideways, mouths directly in front of each other's genitals. When the woman bends the top of her legs at her knee and places her feet flat on the bed, the partners' heads can rest comfortably on each other's thighs.

Some people find it difficult to concentrate on their own pleasure while they focus on their partner. But couples should enjoy the act for the while body touching intimacy it provides. It is an incredibly sexy and intimate way for partners to connect and turn each other on.

Chapter 3: The Evergreen Sex Positions

Missionary Position

The missionary position is one of the simplest and most comfortable positions. It is easy to perform. The woman lies on her back on the bed. Despite its simplicity, this position is one of the most intimate. Couples are close to each other and can kiss and touch each other's bodies during intercourse.

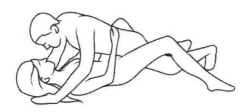

To get into this position, the woman simply lies down, and the man lies on top of her, face down. There is a little difficulty aiming for the man, and it would be helpful for her to help him find her insertion point.

She moves up when he penetrates deep and pulls back at the same moment he pulls back.

This position is pleasing to the woman because the man's body rubs against her clitoris with every thrust he makes. The combination of thrust and clitoral stimulation can help the woman have deep and long orgasms.

The missionary position needs variety to keep it exciting. Hip movements in this position produce surprising sensations because the movement lets the penis contact different areas inside the vagina.

This position is only recommended for couples who know each other well and have been intimate often beforehand. Partners can kiss each other, gaze into each other's eyes while they engage in coitus. There is almost full body contact, another intimate feature of missionary.

Women in general enjoy the missionary position. Aside from allowing them to relax and mostly receive the pleasure from his body moving above her, women have reported that they find it very intimate, and not a position one would do on a first date. Others love the fact that they remain close to their partner, allowing them to kiss each other.

A very nice variation to missionary is when the man mounts her, put penetrates when his body is situated several inches above her. His head is in front of hers (closer to the headboard or end of the bed). His penetration is not as deep, but in exchange, the base of his penis rubs against her clitoris. Her stimulation is greatly increased, and she will feel the impact of his adjustment within seconds. After she comes to a heated orgasm, he can move back into his normal position above her and ejaculate.

The missionary position is one of the most gentle and intimate, but the penis does not go the deepest it can, although the inherent clitoral stimulation can compensate.

Doggystyle Position

There is something just primal about sex in the doggy style position. Males can get very aggressive and transform "vanilla" intercourse into more intense and rougher sex. Men can thrust hard into their partner, and woman generally love receiving the harder thrusts from her partner. In fact, very few women don't enjoy doggystyle.

There are many reasons why doggystyle is so popular, and it truly warrants the praise it receives from both men and women. The advantages it provides for him is his ability to penetrate deeply, while moving in and out at different speeds. He can start slow but become fast very quickly. Ejaculating in doggystyle position is very satisfying for him, especially when he comes inside her vagina.

Setting up for doggy style is simple. On a yielding surface (pillows are recommended under her knees), females get on all fours while he either stands or kneels behind her. Insertion is relatively easy as her vagina is presented in full view.

She can move her hips back and forth in rhythm with his movement. A nice variation is when he raises her hips a little, changing the angle of penetration, satisfying to both partners. The best part of positions like doggystyle is the ability to alter the angle. Even a little change can cause a marked difference in the sensation. With practice, hip movements can be adjusted until couples find the most satisfying angles together.

One of the downsides to doggystyle is that there is no face to face contact with your lover. On the other hand, it's understood that sacrificing the intimacy of looking at your lover's face is made up for by the enjoyment each partner gets. For men, it's a wonderful way to have harder sex, pleasing himself and his partner. Doggy style allows him to thrust as fast as he wishes, and the faster and deeper his thrusts are, the more his partner enjoys it.

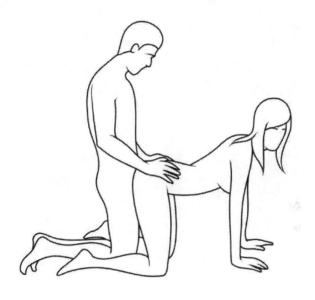

He can pull his partner's hair, smack her buttocks, and even pull her up so her back touches his body and wrapping his arms around her waist. The location of his penis will determine how it touches the G-spot, so couples should experiment with different angles until the spot is reached.

If the tip of his penis makes contact with this area and he is thrusting with a fast speed and still able to thrust deeply at a higher speed, she can have a deep and intense orgasm. She can have several orgasms, in fact.

This position is also good for her if she is able to have vaginal orgasms, because of his depth and the tight friction against her inner vaginal walls.

When starting out, go slowly so each partner can avoid premature orgasm.

Legs Up G-Spot Stimulation

With practice, this position will always stimulate a woman's g-spot, while giving increased pleasure to the man due to the narrower vaginal opening.

The position is different from the woman simply spreading her legs wide for male penetration. Instead, the woman lies on her back and lifts her legs so her feet rest on her partner's shoulders. By doing this, her vaginal opening is narrowed and when the man penetrates, he experiences the pleasure of friction against the woman's vaginal walls.

The narrower opening of the vagina directs his penis directly to her g-spot. As partners practice the position, the woman can ask her partner to rock her body side to side, or, when grasping her thighs, move her up and down while thrusting. Both of these variations will stimulate her deep at her g-spot, giving her different kinds of sensual stimulation.

This is yet another position, where with slight adjustments, he can stimulate the woman and drive her towards an explosive orgasm. The man is in control of movement while she receives, moving her hips while lying on the bed on her back.

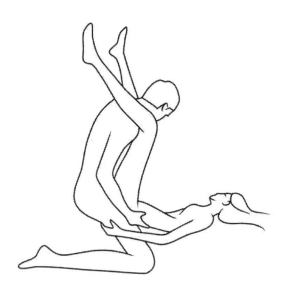

Note that when performing any sexual position involving intercourse, slight movements of the woman's hips, minute changes of angles of penetration, and entering a little higher up and penetrating the vagina from above, can dramatically alter the sensations felt. Trying new positions is experimenting, and when trying, change the angle and move the hips for different stimuli.

Chapter 4: Spooning Sex

Spooning is not only a very comfortable sexual position; it is also incredibly stimulating for several reasons. Couples lie side by side, able to have whatever body contact they desire. Feet, legs, buttocks and back, all can come together.

There are several ways to spoon. The ale enters she from behind, he is raising she's leg if he wishes. Raising a leg allows for deeper penetration. On the other hand, for more body contact, the man can raise her leg and penetrate, and then release it. This results in full body contact, and the feel of skin on skin induces pleasure right along with the thrusts.

Spooning often occurs after couples have been cuddling in bed. Both he and female partners have total access to breasts and clitoris. Spooning is one of the best positions for intimacy. After climax, partners often fall asleep in the position, and awaken hours later with he's penis still inside... and hard. If he's only 50 percent hard, women can just move a little bit and the friction will make him stiffer. A morning quickie in the same position as the night before is a great way to start a day!

There are 4 wonderful variations to spooning.

Woman on Top

Spooning with the female on top is yet another electrifying variation on the normal side to side way of performing spooning. Spooning with her on top still allows for full body contact except it is the woman's back resting on the man's chest and abdomen.

The enjoyment and the intimate feel of spooning is not lost as couples maintain full body contact. He lies supine on the bed and she lies on top of him on her back. He inserts his penis and she feels his thrusts in a unique place inside her vagina, close enough to her G-spot that the tip of his penis can make contact.

This position can be intensely stimulating without requiring a lot of work. For this position, the man lies on the bed or another flat, comfortable surface. The woman is on top. She presses her legs firmly together for a tighter feel. Next, she tilts her pelvis down a little bit, so her clitoris has better contact with the top of her lover's penis.

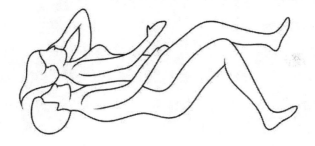

Men can use lube and rub it on his lover's vulva, making smooth hand contact with her clitoris, labia and vaginal opening. He glides his hand up and down her vulva on his out thrusts and moves hand down when he pushes inside.

This position can get even more intimate when the man wraps his arms around her stomach from below, string her nipples and squeezing her breasts. Any additional contact beyond penetration will be arousing to her, and his as well. A woman can achieve both G-spot and vaginal orgasms in this reverse approach.

When she achieves orgasm, it will be simple for her to turn her body over and face him and continue in missionary position. Couples should try to keep his penis inserted while she rotates her body 180 degrees to face him. Sex can be a fun game when couples try to be successful at trails such as these. After all, it is for enjoyment and if his penis can't remain inside her, all he needs to do is to put it back in.

Although she is in a reverse position on top of him, couples should remain relaxed and enjoy the new sensations felt, and revel in the full body intimacy this position offers.

When men reach around, they can increase their lover's pleasure by moving hands down to her clitoris and rub it, wither with or without lube, depending on what she desires. He can reach further down and finger her labia and vaginal opening while he thrusts inside her. This raises intimacy to an even higher level. He has the power to make her scream in erotic pleasure, and from time to time gyrate his hips into her body.

The Nirvana Doggystyle

This method of spooning involves her curling up into herself and then sliding back her feet. For support, he grips her hips.

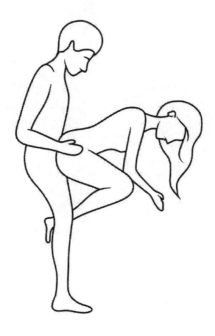

Doggystyle spooning allows for the tip of his penis to reach into infrequently explored nether regions inside her vagina. The friction he experiences from penetration at this unusual angle is highly pleasurable, but the real beneficiary of doggystyle spooning is her, because not only does his penis touch her G-spot, it also reaches other areas that provide unique and unusual sensations.

This spooning position gives intense stimulation to a woman's genitals. She curls her body up as if she herself was a dog. She slides her feet back as he holds on to her hips. This position allows for very deep penetration that's intensely satisfying to her.

The Hard Thrusting

For fast, explosive sex with a lot of deep thrusting, this position is one of the best to achieve a deep and satisfying orgasm for both partners.

This is the most conventional spooning position for couples. It is a nice when used as the final act to a hot, sexual session in the bedroom beginning with 69, followed by Girl on Top, in which she achieves a deeply satisfying orgasm, and Spooning with some good hard thrusting from him, leading to his own orgasm.

It is a comfortable position for her, since she can lie sideways and relaxed while he finishes himself off with penetration from behind. All she needs to do is lift her upper leg and wrap it around behind him and over his buttocks. This allows him to enter through an unusual angle that makes her vagina a little smaller and tighter, and also his thrusts go into her at a different angle in a downward direction.

He props himself up on his elbow behind her, and grabs hold of his partner's thigh, allowing him to make deep, vigorous thrusts that will send shock waves of pleasure through her body.

If she can have vaginal orgasms, then this position can bring it about due to his being able to penetrate her more deeply. With her raised leg, she can reach down and rub her clitoris while he trusts into her.

Women can position themselves near a wall or a headboard and prop a hand against it for leverage. Doing this, she establishes a rhythm with him by pushing into him each time he pushes into her.

Anal Penetration and a Wand

For couples trying anal sex for the first time, this is a great position that prevents too hard and too deep (and painful) penetration into the anus. The man isn't on his partner, which prevents him from going too deep.

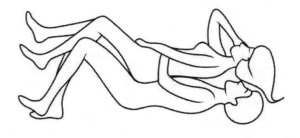

Partners are advised to use lube to coat the penis and the entrance to the anus. They should also go very slowly until reaching a threshold of speed and depth. A woman trying this spooning position can make it more sensually stimulating by using a curved metal wand to insert into her vagina at the same time her partner penetrates her anally.

She rocks the wand gently inside her vagina, matching his thrusts. One of the wonderful surprises that comes from using the wand is that her partner feels it when he penetrates anally.

Chapter 5: Spicy Sex Positions

Seated Cowgirl

This position requires a chair that the man sits upon and his female partner mounts him, straddling his legs on the chair. The Seated Cowgirl position can be performed anywhere a chair can be placed. It can even be performed during a shower if the chair is waterproof.

She lowers herself onto her lover's hard erection (the position will not work unless his penis is fully engorged and stiff). The woman's body is close to her lover's so her feet may touch the ground straddling him.

She should have decently strong thighs, because she'll want to gyrate up and down on her lover's penis. Go slowly and work up speed.

If you try the Seated Cowgirl in the shower, use the shower ledge for support. The couple will want to try the man's penis penetrating both vaginally and anally. Silicon lube is advised for anal sex.

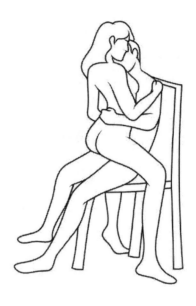

The bodies of each partner are very close to each other. As the woman rides on top, she gyrates her hips. He can wrap an arm around her back and pull her closer, sucking on her breasts and biting her nipples, all while deeply penetrating her. She rides his penis buried deep inside her and rocks to a deep and intense orgasm.

Man on Top

The Man on Top position can be considered a sort of reverse missionary. The difference is that the physical sensations are more intense. Male penetration goes much deeper in this position, and for the woman, his penis size feels much larger than it is.

For any man who loves viewing his lover's buttocks (and even smacking them with glee from time to time), this position provides great sexual release for both partners.

Females lie face down on the bed, and slightly raise their hips. Her lover penetrates her from above, often by kneeling, although with practice, he can make full body contact (reverse missionary). Her partner presses his palms onto the bed to maintain his position. He thrusts into her.

For a sensuous variation, the man can press into the woman's back (while raising up his upper body and pressing down gently. With is hands free, he can slap the woman's butt, run his hands underneath and stroke and squeeze her breasts.

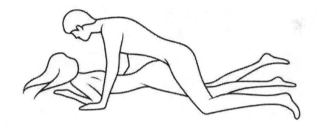

His penis feels larger and the sensation is unique for her. With practice, she can move her pelvis into his in rhythm with his thrusts. By doing so, she can navigate the tip of his penis towards her g-spot.

When he ejaculates inside, to both partners it feels like semen goes deeply inside. Females can take note of the different sensations of his ejaculate in her body.

Man on Top is a sensuous position that gives erotic pleasure which both partners enjoy. When coitus starts with the missionary position, after a while she can flip her body over and he penetrate her on top, with a completely different set of sensations for him and her.

Face to Face Woman on Top

This position is a variation of the seated cowgirl position above, in that this is a more relaxed and comfortable position. This face to face position is more intimate and allows for greater movement of both partner's hands.

This face to face position can be attempted on the edge of a bed, on a couch or a chair. If the bed has a headboard, the man can rest his back against it while his partner sits on top of him.

The man is sitting up and the woman sits on top of him, so they're face to face. He penetrates her and she rocks up and down on top of him. Hands free, she can run her hands over her breasts and stroke her clitoris as his thrusts move deep inside her.

He has the freedom to run his hands all over her body, breasts and back. He can reach forward and bite her nipples. He can take hold of her arms and then wrap his arms around her back to draw her close to him to embrace.

His penis goes deeper in this position. A great advantage is that his orgasm is delayed due to the angle of penetration. Females can indulge in the enjoyment because the position is comfortable and can be maintained for a long time.

It is the kind of position that, because it's so intimate, partners who know each other well, and are comfortable with each other, would want to do. It would not be a position to do with someone unfamiliar, or someone whom you just met. Couples can touch each other, kiss, stroke each other's bodies affectionately and please each other in ways they know their partner loves. A date or one-night meetup would be awkward.

The man can raise the intensity of the position by lifting up the woman's buttocks with his hands and legs and grip them hard, separating their bodies from each other a little. Kissing each other, the feel of the penetration feels more intense, and it raises the temperature, creating more passion.

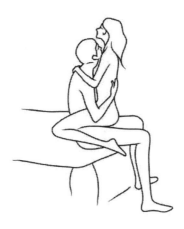

During intercourse, many couples underestimate the erotic sensations that come from touching and shows of affection during coitus. The may not even realize that the touching stimulates nerve endings at the location of body contact and stimulates the genitalia at the same time.

Never underestimate the value of showing tender affection while thrusting harder and harder into her vagina. It may seem like partners are conveying two different sentiments at the same time, tenderness and intense movement, but mastering this juxtaposition will virtually assure orgasms for each partner, some of them coming with greater intensity, while at the same time cementing their affection for each other.

Standing and Facing

Having intercourse while standing up is usually completed when the man stands behind the woman and enters her in that manner. Standing and facing each other and penetrating is still another intimate position for partners because they are able to embrace and look into each other's eyes during penetration.

Partners who have great affection for each will love this position, though it requires some practice to master it. Once it's done right, it provides yet another way to have intercourse, and married or long-term partners can put the position on their list of accomplishments.

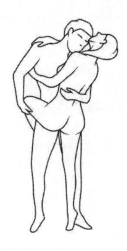

To perform the Standing and Facing Position, the woman stands on one leg and wraps the other around her partner's waist, who holds it during the act. The raised leg is necessary for penetration. The feeling of the friction will be dramatically different. The real purpose of the position is for each partner is to have quality face time.

Facial recognition while bodies are connected through the penis inside the partner, the two can watch each other's facial expressions and register how every different movement stimulates the other. This is one of the highest levels of intimacy. Getting to know how your lovemaking affects the other is getting to understand your partner on a much deeper level.

The Wheelbarrow

The Wheelbarrow sex position is a male-dominant position, allowing him to feel the deepest penetration into his partner. It is a variation of doggystyle and requires some arm strength and endurance from the woman who performs this position.

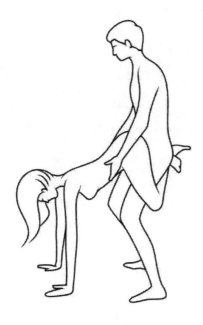

First, she gets on her hands and feet (instead of hands and needs in doggystyle). He lifts her up by her pelvis. She wraps her legs and feet around his waist and thighs.

Holding her by the pelvis, he penetrates her, first feeling the sensation of depth. It is stimulating for his penis to go deeper inside her. He controls the sex act, leaving her to keep her hands planted on the ground and legs up, as the man thrusts inside of her, executing complete control.

Chapter 6: Kinky Sex Positions and Sexual Role Playing

Nothing is better that slicing things up a bit in the bedroom... and being open to trying new things. When there is that spark of physical chemistry between partners, then anything they try will likely be hot and satisfying.

On the other side and out of the light is another world of pleasure and unique approaches to sex and the ways people derive satisfaction from it. On the other side are people who experience and enjoy bondage and role playing. People involved in BDSM sexuality report experiencing deeper levels of pleasure that is highly intense. In their "scenes," sexual role-playing encounters, a partner teases and inflicts moderate to extreme levels of pain upon the other, deriving intense sexual satisfaction when pain is inflicted and from a state of discomfort, achieve a state of serenity and peacefulness.

But not everything in BDSM has to do with pain. Teasing and delaying or denying climax as long as possible, making it build and build without immediate release, makes for explosive orgasms.

In role playing, one partner acts as the dominant who is in control of the sexual activities. The other is a submissive, who is restrained and under the dominant's control and his every whim. Both enjoy these roles tremendously, and sometimes even switch roles. In this case, she can be dominant while he submits to her control. Since it's a role playing, everything is agreed upon at the start, and if things get rough, submissives recite a "safe word" to stop the teasing or discomfort.

When doing role-playing scenarios, it's best that your partner is someone you can trust and with whom you know well and feel safe. For those who are curious, what follows are a few sex positions you may want to try with a kink-minded partner who wants to get a taste of something completely different. You may find you like the experience and if so, can access most anywhere other ideas and go to more thrilling extremes.

Kidnapped and Tied to the Bed

You've been abducted and somehow you went unconscious. You wake up and find that you are naked, and you can't move. You don't know where you are, and what's worse, you're blindfolded. You hear voices somewhere outside the door.

Now you hear footsteps coming closer, and the sound of a door opening. Your captor is in the room with you. Your panic as your heart begins to race. You try again to move, but your ankles and wrists are in restraints. What does he want with you?

This sex position has her on the bed in soft, comfortable cuff restraints. She can either be blindfolded or not. The bottom line is, she's completely under the control of her partner, who can do with her whatever he wishes.

The Tied to the Bed sex position begins with sexual teasing, leading to hot and steamy sexual intercourse when the submissive partner ultimately gets her satisfaction. The dominant partner (in this case, him, although roles can easily be reversed), can use an assortment of "toys" such as a tickler wand to apply to her vagina and clitoris.

If she is blindfolded and tied to the bed, the dominant partner can either talk to her and tell her what he is doing, or he can surprise her. Terms can be set prior to beginning the scene.

However, going blindfolded adds excitement, because the partner who is tied doesn't know what her partner is going to do next. Not knowing builds anticipation and sexual excitement and is teased in such a way that seeing wouldn't allow for.

He can kiss her in expected places or change the way he touches her. She won't know where her partner's mouth and fingers will be next. The dominant partner can come and go as he pleases, building anticipation further. He can assume a different voice, and if he's really creative, play the part of a complete stranger, which will raise her excitement to new heights. As the brain releases cortisol and adrenaline, it also stimulates the body, releasing high levels of dopamine, and the feat becomes combined with pleasure after a period of time.

In more extreme cases, it can turn into a consensual BDSM scenario. The partner can slap the submissives vagina, resulting in some pain followed by pleasure. Leave the room for a period of time, return and repeat the slap. After a time she will anticipate with hot desire your next slap.

When the anticipation becomes unbearable, she begs for release, you can untie her and engage in intense, passionate lovemaking. After both of you have climaxed, the dominant partner brings her down with caresses and other shows of physical affection.

In the Hot Seat - Woman is Dominant

Imagine one day you caught your male lover eyeing another woman, his eyes focused on her just a second too long. Sure, men do watch women walking, bending over, smiling and showing their cleavage all the time. But now it's time he learns the less that what he's got now is a thousand percent hotter and sexier than everyone he fantasized about.

You tell him to sit down on a specially prepared chair you made ready just for him. He knows you want to punish him for being naughty in some way or another, so he plays along.

The moment he's seated, you order him to put his arms behind his back. He does so and you promptly tie his wrists together with some rope you had handy. By his ankles you have more rope, and you bind his ankles promptly to the chair legs.

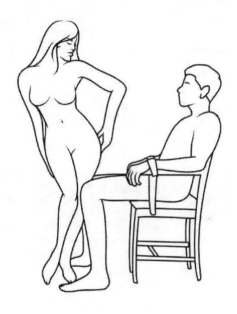

He sits there confused and maybe just a little bit scared. You start asking him about the women he was looking today when the two of you were out. He defends himself, saying he couldn't help it, the way they were dressed and how they teased him and all...

You walk close to him and lean forward, as if you were about to plant a kiss on his lips. At the last moment you draw back and walk over to the music player and turn in on. One of your favorite songs play, the kind strippers dance to in the topless clubs. You remove one article of clothing, then another, really slowly. And you walk towards him, but you're just out of reach.

You watch him eyeing you breasts, hips, legs and as you remove more clothing, and it turns you on. You look down and see his bulge, and you get a little hotter. Finally, standing naked, you let him stare at you, horny and helpless to do anything about it because he's tied up.

You keep him tied and unzip his pants, pulling out his throbbing shaft and you mount him. He can't do it, so you take the tip and put it inside of you, letting it glide down all the way to the stem. You rock up and down on hit as he watches you but can't touch you and you thrust yourself up and down until you reach and screaming, intensely satisfying orgasm at his expense.

Then you untie him and pull him into the bedroom to finish him off.

In this role-reversal scenario, his legs are tied to the chair legs and his arms to the chair arms. Or, his wrists can be secured together behind the chair back. The dominant will begin teasing her male captive.

She can get him thoroughly worked up with a slow striptease, raising his desire for you to a level of slight discomfort and frustration. Next, stroke yourself, masturbate in front of him. Your soft moans will drive him wild, as he tries to get out of is restraints.

Continue to masturbate until you're close to orgasm and he can barely take it any longer. Wait for him to beg. Wait a little longer. Make him beg a little more. Wait a few moments, then mount him. Straddle the chair with your legs and have your way with him on top. Both of you will end up having explosive orgasms.

The man restrained on the chair sees his lover displaying a different, dominant personality, which is itself a turn on for him. It suggests to him that he is with a stranger which releases endorphins in his brain which increase his desire for his female partner tremendously.

Chapter 7: Passionate and Sensual Sex Positions

Passionate Propeller

This position is an erotically charged variation of the missionary position. It should be noted that this is a more advanced sexual position, requiring the partner to move 360 degrees over his female partner lying underneath.

This position allows each partner to feel new and sensual stimulation from the movement of the penis, coming into contact with different areas inside the vagina. The partner on top also benefits from the erotic sensations as he explores inside and feels unique contact in the vagina's nether regions.

He begins in the missionary position above his lover. He penetrates and remains in missionary as each partner works up close to orgasm. But beforehand, he begins a 360-degree spin, all the while keeping his penis deep inside. As he rotates and thrusts, from underneath she helps him in his rotation, the challenge being to keep the penis deep and thrusting all the while.

The woman grabs hold of his thighs and arms as she guides him around, rewarded with the deep thrusts into her as she tries to focus on moving is body around on top of her.

Reverse Cowgirl

Reverse cowgirl is exactly what its title says — the cowgirl position, or woman on top, except instead of her facing her partner as she rides him from above, she reverses her body, now with her back and butt facing him as she looks away.

This is a woman in control position, allowing her to move above her male partner using her arms, knees and hips. She can do whatever feels best to her. Women can play around with motions and angles, move up and down, grind in circles back and forth. She can flex her back which allows her male partner's member to come into contact with her most sensitive internal areas. Females have access to their clitoris, so she can play with it or press it down into her partner's body. If she chooses, she can add a vibrator for more intense stimulation.

If he wants to get involved as she responds to his thrusts, he can wrap his arm around her midsection and pull her back a little towards him as he continues his deep thrusts. He will find this angle gives him intensely pleasurable sensations, as well as his partner. He can release his control and let her once again control the movement.

She can find, if she arches her back backwards towards her partner's head, that her G-spot is touched by the tip of his penis. Like rubbing her clit with her finger, an up and down motion of her body in this backward angle will produce a deep and intense sensation she may have not felt ever before

To perform the Reverse Cowgirl, he lies on his back as she assumes the position on top of him. Facing away from him, she inserts his penis. She steadies herself on the bed with her legs, using her other hand to keep the base of his penis steady.

The Reverse Cowgirl can also be performed on the edge of the bed, in a chair or on the sofa. Here she eases herself down on his lap. Performing the position this way takes the added challenge of remaining balanced out of the realm of possibility. She is more comfortable and can explore movements and test how they feel to her.

Once she's been satisfied, she can lie on her side for her partner to spoon her and achieve orgasm, or fall onto her back, spent and satisfied, while he thrusts into her in missionary until he ejaculates.

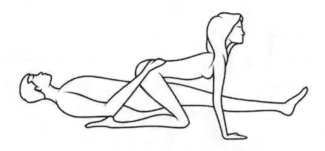

This is a great position for the woman to learn to be in control. It is easy for her to learn to navigate over her partner's body and by adjusting her angle, change the sensation response, and when repeated often, the Reverse Cowgirl will allow the woman to learn for her experience and eventually find the most erotically arousing angle of her partner's penetration. Any anxiety she feels at the start will fade away over time.

One of the wonderful things about trying new sex positions is how much partners can learn from working through many different ones. Lovers find out along the way that all their original beliefs about sex, specifically the belief that orgasm and sexual arousal feels one way and one way only, are blown out the window as each new position opens vistas of sexual pleasure never felt before.

The Piledriver

The Piledriver sexual position requires couples have a good deal of flexibility. However, with some repetitive practice, the position becomes much easier. One of the benefits of the position is that it permits both vaginal sex and anal sex to be performed.

When setting up for the position, the woman lies on her back, then lifts up her legs in the air. Her male partner grabs her legs by the back of her ankles and pushes them toward the woman's head. Her lower back will lift up off the bed. Ideally, he will keep pushing her ankles forward towards her head until her entire back is off the bed (or ground). All that should remain on the bed are the woman's shoulders and the back of her head.

All the women need do in this position is to hold herself steady while the man penetrates. She does this by putting her arms on the ground or bed, or by grabbing and holding on to the man's ankles. Females in the Piledriver position find how easy it is for them to masturbate (if they have long enough arms). This intensifies her sexual experience.

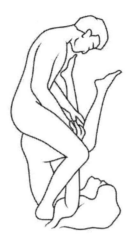

The man does most of the work in this position. He needs to keep she steady while he penetrates at the same time. When engaging in vaginal sex, the man can use his hands to rub her clitoris. If engaging in anal sex, he can finger her clit and vagina while anally penetrating her.

NOTE: Another way to get into this position is to sit down on a sofa backwards, the opposite of normal. Her back and waist are supported by the backrest while her shoulders and head are where her buttocks normally are. She may find this position far more comfortable.

Female Launch and Curl

The Launch and Curl position is an extremely pleasurable position for her and has the pleasant feeling of him being on top of her, in a dominant position. If neither partner has tried this position, it comes here highly recommended.

To get into the Launch and Curl position, she lies on her back. The male, facing her, penetrates her while on his knees and facing her. She lifts her legs upwards and brings her knees to her chest, curling her body. Then her feet rests on his chest. He can then lean over her, which allows her to raise her hips us easily. This allows for very deep penetration from him.

When she lies on her back in the Launch and Curl position, her male partner will seem to appear as if he has most of the control. However, she will have the most. Because her feet are on his chest, she controls how deep his penetration can go. She can adjust and make the penetration shallow or deep.

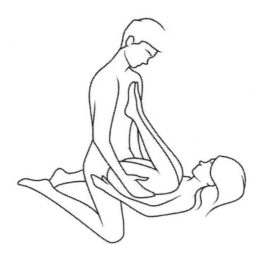

If uncomfortable, she can always put her feet on either side of him or move both to one of his sides. As her hips are slightly lifted, she can masturbate herself to a satisfying orgasm.

The Launch and Curl position is comparatively easier and more straightforward for the man. He only needs to thrust in and out. If she wants to be penetrated at a different angle, one that yields G-spot stimulation, then he will need to adjust himself a little bit. He moves from leaning over and moves back and away until reaching the right angle for G-spot contact.

Anal sex can be attempted in this position as well.

Hanging Garden

This position is highly sensual for both partners, because it is intimate and at the same time somewhat more rough than other sex positions. Doing the Hanging Garden sex position is great for a man with strong arms and a petite woman, or a strong man and a woman who is larger.

To perform this position, the man literally lifts the woman off the ground and holds her. She wraps her legs around him a little above his waist. He penetrates while holding her secure in his arms.

The man thrusts his body forward as he penetrates the woman. Her arms are wrapped around his neck for support. Their faces are very close. They can kiss as his penis glides in and out of her vagina. While this position requires the man to have strength and be fit, it is also intensely intimate. When sexual arousal rises, the female's body feel lighter, and the man's arms feel as if they are not holding any weight at all. Intimacy and erotic pleasure take over, and even the female forgets she is being held.

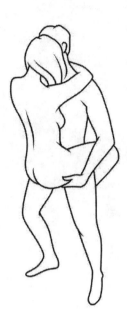

Kneeling Sex Position

Being able to look at each other during intercourse only makes intercourse that much better. Positions like Kneeling Sex is yet another very intimate shared experience as lovers look into each other's eyes while their bodies experience intense states of arousal.

. They can look at each other, kiss, embrace and press their bodies together. They are also in an upright position off the bed, which adds even more excitation.

To get into the kneeling position, her partner stands on the floor. She kneels on the bed, facing him. Make sure the base of the man's penis is at about the same height as the woman's vaginal opening. If an adjustment needs to be made, place a few sturdy, hardcover books under the bed to raise it up, or he can stand on something and adjust until penetration is possible.

What the Woman does in the Kneeling Position

Women will not get a lot of pleasure by remaining upright throughout. For better stimulation, she should lean backwards. In this way, her partner can support her, and she can put her hands around his waist. If she wishes to lean back further, she can place her hands behind her on the bed. If her partner is holding her, or if she is using one hand for support, she's easily able to rub her clitoris with her free hand.

For men, watching a woman masturbating is a major turn on. In this way, he watches and gets aroused while the woman pleasures herself.

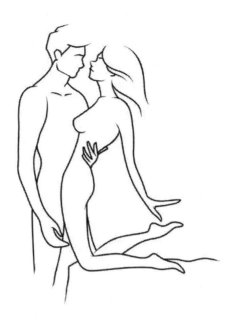

The Man's Role in the Kneeling Position

He has little to do in this position while his female partner is kneeling on him. He only needs to get in the best possible position to make deep and satisfying thrusts. As mentioned before, he can do more by supporting her atop him. For additional stimulation, the man can spank the woman as she pleasures herself.

When she is in the upright position, he can kiss and hold close his female partner. But if she is leaning back, he can put his hands on her breasts and rub them and gently swirl her nipples, not too hard to take away from her bodily stimulation, but only enough to enhance her pleasure.

Chapter 8: Anal Sex Position

Even with our modern-day sentiment of openness and acceptance, sex involving the area around the buttocks is still one of the most divisive sex acts. There are those who really, really love it. And there are those on the opposite end of the spectrum, who really hate it. But people who are curious won't really know what side of the fence they're on until they try it for themselves.

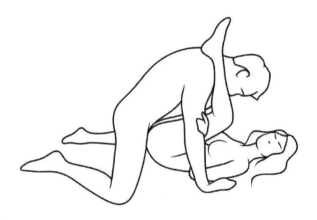

Preparing for anal sex requires a woman to lubricate her anus, and for the best experience, relax the muscles there for the best experience. Unlike a vagina, the rectum doesn't lubricate itself. Anal intercourse may seem intimidating for a novice. If women take their time with anal foreplay (fingering and rimming), the odds of enjoying it are a lot better.

Preparation for Beginners:

- Get a water-based lubricant. This will make rubbing and massaging even better. Even if foreplay doesn't involve any fingers penetrating, lubricant makes improvement in the area and can also increase sensitivity.

- Use some female sex toys to get the process going. A vibrating toy with a broad head is recommended. Place the head of the vibrator against the anal opening but don't insert it. Run it in a circle around the opening. External anal vibrations add completely new sensations. Alternate between the vibrator and your finger to start teasing yourself into getting ready.

- Women have partners give them a buttocks massage. Start off with a sensual massage of the buttocks. Using lube, he places his thumbs in the creases at the point where the legs meet the butt cheeks and slide the thumbs along the crease form the inner thigh area to the outer side. Lift, then repeat. Next, put the palms together, as if one is praying, and press down on the tailbone of your partner. Move on, gliding the hands up and down the butt crack.

- When he penetrates, it should not hurt. She should only feel like she has to go, but she doesn't. Relax the muscles of the anus and breathe.

- She could test first to see if she will like it by trying it out on her own first. Place an index finger inside and insert the length of the finger. Although it won't be the same as your partner penetrating with his penis, she will still know if she enjoys the sensation.

- Try it out in the bathtub first. Being in warm water relaxes the muscles and is a great place to determine if you will like it. If there's any concern about cleanliness (not a real issue), your fears can be allayed. Plus the pressure of his penis inside you is made easier the first time by the water.

- Your partner should err on the shallow side the first time. Penetrating and thrusting like a man would with vaginal sex, he should go much slower and no thrust too deeply into her.

- Anal sex is not dirty, as medical doctors state that there is very little or no fecal material in the area, so if couples are thinking about doing anal sex, don't take this into account.

- Anal sex is most enjoyable when there is other stimulation happening at the same time. Vaginal, clitoral and nipple rubbing, or friction will enhance the experience. Prior to the first time, she should empty her bowels, then shower and clean the area well.

The Posterior Anal

The woman lies face down on the bed completely extended. The man mounts her from above and his body is also fully extended. He presses down on the bed with the palms of his hands for support on either side of her. He penetrates slowly into the woman's anus.

Both partners are very relaxed in this easygoing position. The woman experiences the least amount of penetration in this position because of the angle of the thrust.

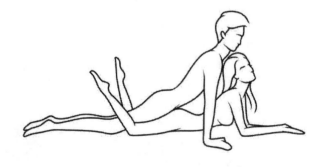

Standing Together Position

The woman stands in front of her partner. And the man penetrates her from behind, both of you standing up. He can reach over your body as he penetrates and squeeze your breasts, twirl your nipples and rub her clitoris to give her extra sensation.

Doggy Style Anal Sex

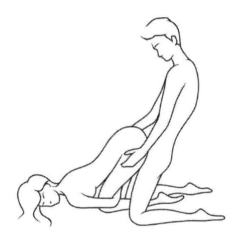

This is the same position as doggy style, except the man inserts his penis into his partner's anus. Again, he can reach down and rub her clit as he moves his hands from her hips.

He can move his hands all over her body as partners assume the most comfortable position for doggystyle, like on a mattress.

Chapter 9: Lotus Sex Position

Regular Lotus Position

The Lotus Position is perfect for intimate couples who know each other well and who want to share an erotic experience together. Couples look at each other face to face as their entire bodies come into contact throughout intercourse in the position, they both rise to orgiastic climax by performing this ancient coupling position.

The man sits down with his legs crossed and the woman straddles him, wrapping her legs around his waist. Next, the couple wrap their arms around each other as if they were hugging. He inserts and penetrates up inside of her from below.

There are few positions that come close to the Lotus for intimacy that leads to affectionate touching and helps enhance closeness in a couple. Kissing and embracing are natural to do in this position.

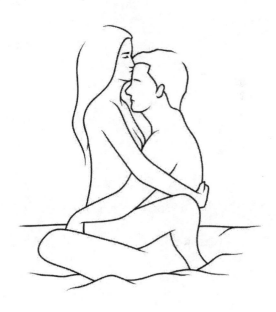

Because of the angle of entry, he can thrust in either an up and down motion or thrust back and forth. A woman capable of internal orgasms would find it easy achieving one when his thrusting penetrates from four different angles.

If the woman on top is finding it difficult to find a good rhythm or range of motion, she can grasp a headboard or put her hands on a wall for anchoring support to help with moving. If this doesn't work, she can unwrap her legs and kneel over her partner like she would in the cowgirl position.

Reverse Lotus

Although this will change the position from lotus to sitting in reverse cowgirl, it's a great variation and there is still an enormous amount of skin to skin contact. Bodies contacting, no matter if it's face forward or backward, is always intimate and warm.

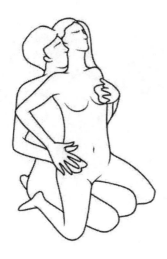

The man sits on a chair or the bed cross legged, and the woman sits on top of him. Couples wrap their arms around each other and enjoy the closeness while he penetrates her, and she feels the erotic intensity grow while she kisses and embraces her partner.

Light Bondage Lotus

Couples can use silk ties to tie up to each other for an added sense of closeness.

Fasten either one or both the hands together and then one partner wraps his arms around the other, so there is the sensation of being bound together.

Chapter 10: Bath Shower Sex Positions

Everyone has at one point in their lives, thought about having sex in the shower. Combined with hot water and soap, shower sex can be intense and memorable, and a great way to add variety to a couple's sex life.

However, shower sex is not easy to pull off until one gains experience doing it. Showers can be cramped, making it logistically difficult, if not impossible. However, for those with large shower stalls, it's definitely worth the extra effort.

Wraparound Shower Sex

Here, the female leans back against the shower wall while her male partner stands in front of her. Next, she wraps one leg around his waist, or he holds the back of her knee in the cork of his elbow.

From this angle, he penetrates her, and because both face each other, he can rub his fingers against her clitoris as he thrusts inside her. For variety, he can use an underwater vibrator.

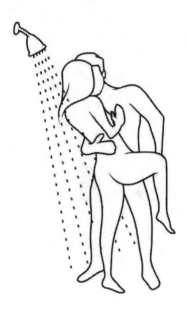

Once it feels normal and under control, couples can do any number of things to each other. They can kiss, the woman can stroke the man's testicles, and he can bend and lick and bite her nipples.

The position works because the female has support from both the wall and from her partner's arms, ensuring neither partner will fall. This is yet another face to face sexual position and looking down to see him penetrating her is a turn on for both partners.

Standing Doggystyle Sex

The female presses her palms against the shower wall and leans toward it at a 45-degree angle. Her knees ae slightly bent for comfort. He can then penetrate her from behind and reach his arm around to play with her clitoris or her breasts, or both.

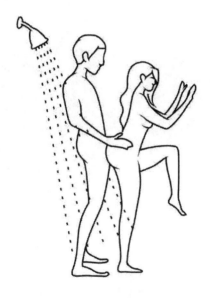

Adding a wash during sex can make it interesting. He has access to her back and can use a sponge to gently rub over her clitoris at the same time.

The female is secure in this position, between the wall and her partner, leaving her free to focus entirely on the sensation without worrying about slipping.

Sitting and Sliding Shower Sex

The male sits on the shower tub's base with his legs stretched out. The woman straddles him from above in any position she chooses.

He can move his body around with greater ease than in bed, so there will be different angles of penetration.

The feeling for her as the hot water pulsates down her back while being penetrated adds to the erotic sensations of this and all shower positions.

She can also control the pace and intensity of his thrusts.

Conclusion

The Human Body and Sexual Sensitivity

There is research that explains why orgasms for both partners occur more easily in the Lotus Sex Position. The body has dozens of erogenous zones that couples may not be aware of, until they begin to experiment with new positions, and discover, to their great surprise, that they feel sensations they never thought possible before.

Organs such as lips, for example, have thousands of nerve endings. Kisses are such a turn on because every part of their surface comes alive when contact is made with them. The rest of the body also has areas in which there are clusters of nerve endings.

The clitoris has 8 thousand nerve receptors, as does the frenulum (the part of the penis known as the glans, which is just under rthe tip of the penis). During penetration, males feel this area stimulated, and the more friction against the frenulum there is, the closer he comes to climax.

The lips are said to be the most sensitive part of the body, with fingertips a close second. This is why when we touch intimately, we are stimulated not just from being touched, but from the act of touching itself.

When couples perform the 69 position, for example, their sensitive lips are moving over sensitive parts of their lover's body, which is why the experience is so stimulating and enjoyable. The neck responds to light touch, the nipples and the clitoris are the most sensitive to pleasure, and the marginal areas of the vagina are also highly sensitive areas.

But there are other areas on a woman, when touched or stroked gently, respond with feelings of sexual pleasure. These include behind the ears, the buttocks and the inner thighs. But what about if a woman hears a deep vibration inside her ear? Does she also have a sexual response?

The answer is yes, if the one speaking into her ear and making the tiny hairs in her ear vibrate is someone she is already attracted to, and who she cares about. On the other hand, if it is a stranger, she neither knows nor trusts, she most likely won't have a sexual response.

What about men? One of the most sensitive areas on a man is under his chin, second only to his penis. A man's neck, lower abdomen and inner thighs are as sensitive as a woman.

Were lovers to keep in mind the primary areas of stimulation, they would soon discover others after trying more sexual positions. For example, a woman is also sensitive under her knees at the crook. Then there are those whose feet, when tickled, generate a sexual response.

In truth, while there is a fixed amount of erogenous body zones, there are differences found in every person. Spending time with a partner, getting to know them sexually, can lead to more intense arousal states during sex. These areas are discovered when trying new sex positions.

Made in United States
Orlando, FL
29 June 2025